Dom's Guide To BDSM Vol. 1

49 Must-Know Tips On How To Be The Perfect Dom/Master Your Submissive Will Truly Respect & Admire

Matthew Larocco

Copyright© 2015 by Matthew Larocco

Dom's Guide to BDSM Vol. 1

Copyright© 2015 Matthew Larocco
All Rights Reserved.

Warning: The unauthorized reproduction or distribution of this copyrighted work is illegal. No part of this book may be scanned, uploaded or distributed via internet or other means, electronic or print without the author's permission. Criminal copyright infringement without monetary gain is investigated by the FBI and is punishable by up to 5 years in federal prison and a fine of $250,000. (http://www.fbi.gov/ipr/). Please purchase only authorized electronic or print editions and do not participate in or encourage the electronic piracy of copyrighted material.

Publisher: Enlightened Publishing

ISBN-13: 978-1517620202

ISBN-10: 1517620201

Disclaimer

The Publisher has strived to be as accurate and complete as possible in the creation of this book. While all attempts have been made to verify information provided in this publication, the Publisher assumes no responsibility for errors, omissions, or contrary interpretation of the subject matter herein. Any perceived slights of specific persons, peoples, or organizations are unintentional.

This book is not intended for use as a source of legal, business, accounting or financial advice. All readers are advised to seek services of competent professionals in the legal, business, accounting, and finance fields.

The information in this book is not intended or implied to be a substitute for professional medical advice, diagnosis or treatment. All content contained in this book is for general information purposes only. Always consult your healthcare provider before carrying on any health program.

Table of Contents

Introduction 5

Chapter 1: How Did BDSM Start? 11
  Domination—A Human Thing 12
  Pain and Pleasure 13
  Sadomasochism 15
  A History of BDSM 16

Chapter 2: Misconceptions About the Dynamic and Lifestyle 19
  Secrets and Lies 21
  Primary and Secondary Masochism? 22
  Who's Really in Control? 23
  Teasing and Delaying 27

Chapter 3: The Difference Between Abuse and Dominance 31
  Patterns of Doms and subs 32
  Patterns by Abusers and Masochists 34
  The Effects of a BDSM Master-Slave Relationship 36

Chapter 4: The Role of the Master 41
    Daddy Loves Who He Disciplines............. 42
    What Do YOU Want Out of This?.............. 43
    What is Leadership?..................................... 46

Chapter 5: The Role of the Slave 51
    What Does the Sub Expect You To Do? 55
    Power Trade 56
    Honesty Shapes Your Master's Thinking Process 58

Chapter 6: The Wrong Way To Do BDSM..... 61

Chapter 7: What Creates a Personal Taboo? . 69
    How Much of Erotic Desire is Social? 73

Chapter 8: Learning Yourself and the Sub's Limits 77
    Being True to Yourself 79
    Keeping it (Not) Real 82
    The Agreement Phase 84
    The Debriefing Phase 85

Chapter 9: Creating Gut Level Attraction by Unleashing Your Passions 87
    How Does the Master Guide the Scene? ... 90

The Importance of Practice 92

Chapter 10: BDSM as Surrogate Therapy...... 97

Conclusion 103

Introduction

BDSM, or Bondage and Discipline (BD), Dominance and Submission (DS), Sadism and Masochism (SM), usually produces a strong reaction in a person who has never studied it. Their initial reaction is usually:

- "BDSM is degrading towards women!"

- "That sounds scary!"

Or maybe a more open-minded reaction like:

- "I've heard of it. It sounds intriguing."

- "I really wouldn't know what to do."

And unfortunately, much of what we've "heard" about BDSM and the lifestyle is wrong. Our opinions on this lifestyle and art form are oftentimes shaped by other people who have heard something about it and perhaps embellished it to the point of perpetuating myths. The truth is that BDSM is not degrading towards women, and it's also a concept that you will find is not "scary", but actually:

- Personal and custom-made for your pleasure
- Made with a person's comfort and self-esteem in mind
- Adaptable
- Highly individual in nature and not a "once size fits all"

And even the "pain" that is spoken of is not the type of pain people think it is. They tend to think "pain" as torture and violence, when in actuality, the one being "dominated" wants the pain. They enjoy it.

And believe it or not, that in and of itself doesn't make a person a masochist. Nor is BDSM all about sex. What you will find, the more you learn about the lifestyle, is that it is an art form and a means of expression that actually helps people come to terms with their feelings, their desires and their wants and needs.

Of course, like most people, you're probably thinking, "I'd rather be a Master than a slave." Because not everyone is thrilled with the idea of being a subordinate.

Not to worry, this book is written for Masters in training. And this book is written for you, the average guy or girl, who doesn't already have a closet full of leather and whips, and who really has no idea what BDSM is besides what they've heard about it.

What you are going to find out though, is that the Master actually has the more complicated role between the two. The master also has the task of giving pleasure and discipline to the slave or sub, and is less focused on taking pleasure himself. A great deal of what you do as a Master will be for the benefit of a sub. You must derive pleasure from giving, and have a great desire to please a partner, and not simply take what you want.

Still interested? Good. Now that we know you're a REAL master in training, one that will respect the rules, respect the slave you have power over, and follow protocol, you can begin your Dom training. In this book we are going to discuss:

- How to think and act like a Dom
- What the slave expects from you
- What not to do and what instincts you do NOT want to follow
- Your motivation and your goals
- How to find out a sub's taboo
- How to negotiate, find agreement and ensure that game play is always safe
- How to make a slave yearn for you and desire to be controlled by you

BDSM has really gone mainstream over the past several years, and it's no coincidence—because people really are looking for sexual fulfillment. Many people today feel unfulfilled sexually, because they have grown accustomed to the routines and really want to spice up their sex life.

And most sources of help stick to the very basics—like changing positions, dressing sexy, exchanging fantasies, and the like.

What you will find about BDSM is that it's far more complex than just "trying something new." It represents a new way of thinking, a new way of acting, and a new hobby that you can take great delight in. Not only because you are living out your fantasy as a Dom who completely controls and satisfies a partner, but also because you will be doing your part to give pleasure to others. Make them feel alive, passionate, excited, and who knows, maybe even help them get over some baggage in their lives.

If you are ready to embrace the lifestyle, and embrace the **instructions** that come along with this training, then by all means keep reading. We're going to go on a personal mission of self-discovery and learn all about the art, hobby and lifestyle of this alternative form of sexuality.

Don't be afraid, it's nothing you can't handle with a little bit of practice, no matter how unsure or introverted you feel right now. Your Master Mentor is here to help you and we're going to make this easy and straight to the point. Let's get started by discussing a little bit about how BDSM got started and what it has evolved to today.

Note: Throughout the book we may use "he" for Dom/Master and "she" for sub/slave. Nevertheless, understand that a Dom/Master can be either male or female, and so can a sub/slave.

Chapter 1: How Did BDSM Start?

BDSM has been around "forever", so to speak, or at least for as long as human beings have learned to "shift the power" in their relationships. Ever since man has developed superior intelligence, he has realized that a master dominating over a lower "class" of slaves has its advantages. And much of that power trip is sexual.

Though today we have outgrown forced slavery as a means to an end, at least in North American and European society, the dynamics of master-slave are still very much alive. With only one real difference: the arrangement is now voluntary. There are no forced slavery arrangements anymore, at least not in respectable and legal BDSM play.

Still, we would be remiss in not going down memory and taking a history lesson about where BDSM comes from—its "shameful" origins in history, because much of the dynamic is based on what we as an intelligence species have already learned.

So our first tip is:

Tip #1: Take the time to read what BDSM actually is. Appreciate that BDSM's origins is purely psychological and thus special attention to history and psychological theory is required.

Domination — A Human Thing

It's important to understand that back when BDSM was first becoming a "thing", way back when, there was no self-awareness, and typically no voluntary arrangement about it. Wealthy families kept slaves, concubines, had multiple wives, and did all sorts of questionable things. Some kings and queens used their slaves as sex toys, for lack of a better word, and fed them aphrodisiacs for the royal nightly orgy — or so they say about Cleopatra.

Obviously, sex was not a game to royals who felt entitled to sex with whomever they wanted, from Jewish King Solomon and his hundreds of wives, to the Emperors of Rome and their notorious debauchery and predilection for public orgies. Therefore, it's safe to assume that much of early master-slave play was involuntary, quite scary, and what we might consider sexual trauma.

Even if BDSM is voluntary nowadays we still retain the illusion of masters "owning" slaves and the *appearance* of total domination. Such as that of a king or emperor, because when a master, a royal speaks, there is no objection.

The master's unquestioning and absolute power is the basis for this relationship, though of course, the dynamic today is a little more complex than Nero or Caligula demanding everyone strip naked for their amusement. Not to worry, we're going to discuss these complexities a bit later. For now, let's talk about old school BDSM, and yes, we really mean old school.

Pain and Pleasure

Long before BDSM was classified by psychology, the concept of pain and pleasure (more or less what BDSM is on an elementary level) was already deeply explored. There are records of the Goddess Inanna, in the B.C. era, that refer to domination rituals, that involved cross-dressing, "pain and ecstasy", initiation proceedings, punishment, "lament and song", weeping and grief and pretty much anything you'd expect to see from a sex dungeon today.

Flagellations (ancient spankings) were on record since at least the ninth century in Artemis Orthia of Sparta, as The Priestess oversaw ritual floggings of young men. These instances, and many more like them, were not merely about the "abuse" of the slave, as in a violent perversion of royalty; but the PLEASURE that such punishment brought both the slave and the master.

Yes, slaves liked it, even if they didn't have much of a choice and even if their master did have all the power and there was no "acting" or "safe word" involved. Because pleasure and pain are always more intense when they accompany each other, as in the words of one very famous novel, "they are on the same scale of human emotion."

The Kama Sutra actually described four types of "hitting" during sex that were to elicit "joyful cries of pain" from bottoms, not tops. In addition, biting, pinching and other forms of impact play were also mentioned. What's interesting is that even in the ancient Kama

Sutra, it is expressed that the sex act should be consensual since not all women would consider it a joyful experience. Therefore, not only did the Kama Sutra realize the reality of pleasure-pain, but it also referred to "rules."

We went from total master-slave power play to a very sophisticated system of sexual rites that had to be performed, just so, much in the same specific way as G-spot and clitoral orgasms had to be performed.

Sadomasochism

While some argue that BDSM is a distinctly modern behavior, coming from 18th and 19th century sexuality, and the psychiatric establishment that attempted to classify it, one can't deny that Marquis de Sade was a forerunner of the pleasure-pain scale, and in fact, helped to bring the word "sadism" into the vernacular. Sadism and masochism, from the etymological point of view, do tend to imply non-consent. And anyone who's read Sade probably remembers that in his stories he describes disturbing scenes of rape and emotional pain.

It's obvious why the master enjoys it, but what about the slave enduring the emotional and physical abuse? Further expansion on the slave's side of things comes from Leopold von Sacher-Masoch, who wrote about his fantasies of being dominated by women and actually signed a contract to become a woman's "slave" for a period of months.

So it's abundantly clear, regardless of official BDSM linguistics, pleasure pain is as old as human sexuality itself.

A History of BDSM

The official definition of BDSM didn't arrive until the 1800's when psychiatry and medicine attempted to convert Christian sin into medical diagnoses. *Psychopathia sexualis* was a major turning point, creating concepts of "perversions", while psychiatrist Richard von Krafft Ebing first began writing about sadism and masochism in his books.

Sigmund Freud was another influential mind, and thoroughly described sadism and masochism, tracing them back to improper child development of the psyche. Since Freud considered it a "disease" it's obvious why much of the BDSM community rejects the label, instead thinking of their sexuality as "aesthetic." Therefore, you will notice that much of the BDSM community avoids S&M terminology, since it is linked with Sade, Freud and all the others who described deviancy, and instead refer to the modernized BDSM.

In essence, BDSM advocates claim it is an identity and not a deviation, nor does it have to be psychological impulse at all; rather, choice, and artistic display. To this day, modern psychiatry still tends to classify the recognized BDSM culture as deviant behaviors and personality disorders.

The reason probably being that, much as Freud documented, fetishes develop in childhood. So while Freud may not have been politically correct in calling it a disease, he was onto something in regards development of fetishes, since childhood is where identity is formed.

The problem is that modern psychiatry still tends to group BDSM with abusive relationships. Which brings us to an important point...

BDSM is not abuse and it's not just a game of Master Says. There are layers of complexity to the BDSM lifestyle.

And with such bizarre portraits of the lifestyle in TV and movies—which oftentimes satirizes it, or ridicules or criticizes it, or in the case of that one movie, sensationalizes it, it is very difficult for a newbie to understand how to act, what to do, and what not to do. Not to worry, this is the subject of our next three chapters.

Chapter 2: Misconceptions About the Dynamic and Lifestyle

Actually, understanding or not understanding BDSM goes well beyond definitions of "aesthetics" vs. deviations. The culture is more interested in the discussion of "Do you actually get BDSM?" or is it all just a joke to you?

Because if it's a joke, or trying it is just an excuse to treat your partner like crap, then no, it's not healthy and it's not even going to be very pleasurable for you or your sub. The Caligula-take-all approach to BDSM is an outdated concept and it's actually evolved into more complex characterizations today, rather than just the Overlord commanding his slave.

Tip #2: Accept that BDSM is no laughing matter and it's not a license to be a dick.

Understanding what real BDSM is, means getting the psychology behind it. BDSM is not accurately portrayed in history, certainly not in the context of psychiatry, and definitely not in the mainstream, when it comes to movies and TV shows.

For instance, some of the most common misconceptions include:

- BDSM is all about pain; the master inflicts pain and the slave loves whatever he gives her.

- BDSM is always about sex.

- BDSM is about one partner abusing the other.

- Subs have low self-esteem.

- The dominant controls the submissive. (More on this later)

- BDSM is about hurting someone else and forcing them to cross all taboos.

- It's all about rape or role play rape.

- You have be to a masochist to enjoy it.

- Doms have to play their part perfectly.

- There is no negotiation—only barking orders.

- BDSM is addictive and all about escalating taboos to the point of extremes.

- BDSM is about avoiding romance and intimacy.

- BDSM is for everyone and is 100% safe.

All of these are "wrong" in some way, and the rest of this book will focus on teaching the reality of what the culture and lifestyle is, as distinct from the image of BDSM that has been fed to us by psychiatry and the perception that something must be wrong with the person.

Secrets and Lies

Let's start with more closely analyzing the origins of fetishism, which are, not surprisingly, connected with prostitution. Back in the day, a man did not experiment with his wife. He went to a prostitute to fulfill his darkest desires, to indulge his unmentionable fetishes, and to live in complete denial of what was forbidden outside of the bordello.

So we see one very important point: BDSM is about experimentation, a comfortable shift away from the traditional approach to romance and sex.

Tip #3: Become comfortable with experimentation. Accept that this will be a learning experience and you're not an all-knowing MASTER just because you're joining the BDSM lifestyle. An open mind is more important right now than attitude.

Primary and Secondary Masochism?

Let's go back to Freud for a moment, not to champion him as a BDSM advocate by any means, but instead to analyze some of what the mainstream has wrong about the lifestyle. Freud taught that there were two forms of masochism. Primary, which was complete rejection by a partner (or the "sadist"), and secondary, which was a sort of "feigned rejection" that was more like a charade or roleplay.

Interestingly, this Freudian model still makes sense because it represents extremes in the sub's desires. Primary rejection would involve continuing punishment or denial, and complete rejection of sexual goals; secondary would simply be a system of reward and punishment, in respects, earning the Master's approval with submissive behavior.

However, the primary misconception here is that the masochist wants primary rejection; he/she actually wants acceptance and wants limits and a BDSM relationship based on negotiation, the opposite of primary rejection, which in theory thrives on hurting or chasing away the masochist.

Tip #4: Remember you are not rejecting the sub for being ____, ____ or ____. (Any abusive terms you can think of) That would defeat the entire purpose of having a slave, wouldn't it?

Who's Really in Control?

Furthermore, Krafft-Ebing and Freud both taught that sadism in men was a distortion of male aggression and that all females were basically masochistic in nature, in that they craved dominance by instinct.

One of the most interesting recent commentaries on the subject comes from Havelock Ellis, *Studies in the Psychology of Sex*, who says that sadism and masochism are so closely related, that they are complementary acts of love; pain is inflicted because of love, not abuse. For the pleasure of both giver and receiver.

He also states another little understood secret of the BDSM lifestyle—sadomasochistic activities (distinguished from abusive relationships) involve the "express request of the masochist" who gives the sadist emotional cues and mutually understood signals—in essence prompting and guiding the sadist on how to properly give him pleasure and pain.

Yes, there you have it. The Master's intent is to please the slave. The sub, the submissive, the bottom, ultimately powers the relationship. After all, it is consensual and voluntary, and the only reason a sub would stay in the "control" of a Dom is to experience pleasure/pain in just the way he or she wants.

Tip #5: Your job is to make your slave happy. It's not to break them or bully them into a crying heap of pain. Ultimately, you are giving the sub what the sub wants.

This is in contrast to many misconceptions out there that express, in so many words:

- That the Master is in control because he's an alpha male, aggressive and confident.

- That the billionaire asshole is in control because of his wealth and power, and the woman's role is to put up with all the tests he gives her.

- That a Dom's main intent is to "tame the shrew" and treat her poorly, breaking her spirit and training her to be a good submissive.

All of these are misconceptions because they don't factor in the base foundation that the sub is the primary receiver of pleasure, and is ultimately in control, since he or she always has the choice to walk away and stop "playing."

True, there are definitely exceptions to the rule, but these exceptions are not considered real BDSM lifestyle or activities—they are abusive relationships in action, or the primary "rejection" Freud talked about, where emotional abuse is craved by the individual with low self-esteem. The sort of old school psychological Sade-created sadism that is addictive and self-destructive and ultimately exhausting.

In contrary, BDSM has the capacity to be aesthetic and what you might call sustainable, in that it doesn't escalate to the point of addiction, nor are there withdrawal pains or "tolerance" that demands constant extremes. It is simply a type of role play, not always sexual in nature, that gives both lovers pleasure without personal manipulation.

Tip #6: Make this play sustainable, repeatable and easy to pick up where you left off.

You are not trying to take your slave to extremes. You are not trying to trespass on your sub's comfort zones, escalating the anxiety. You are trying to have them keep coming back.

Teasing and Delaying

In keeping with the same Freudian dissection, secondary rejection is clearly at play in real BDSM, since ultimately the sub gets the stimulation he wants. He/she just doesn't get it right now. The Master has the task of increasing frustration and delaying the sub's desire for gratification.

French philosopher Gilles Deleuze wrote on masochism, and describes one of the more subtle pleasures of the dance; the masochist gets pleasure from the contract of the arrangement. Delaying release, sexual or non-sexual gratification, either intensifies the sub's feelings when orgasm is imminent, or completely denies gratification altogether, by creating a loop of delay and teasing—which the sub finds orgasmically gratifying in and of itself.

The sub controls the Master, turning the Master into someone "cold, callous"; while the sadist tries to "destroy the ego, unify the id and super-ego" and thus satisfy BASE desires. While this isn't exactly the principle of BDSM, it is true that the sub ultimately decides the future of the relationship and the Master becomes the role the sub wants.

For now, let's review the most basic lessons of BDSM lifestyle:

- It is about experimentation and negotiation
- The sub always has control even if the appearance is that the Master does
- The sub wants to be teased and the Master knows how to delay and pleasantly torture and deprive the sub to his/her heart's content

QUESTION: Is Fifty Shades of Grey an accurate portrayal of BDSM lifestyle?

ANSWER: Tricky question, because although the book and the movie does speak of the lifestyle and uses some common scenarios found in BDSM, it is not technically following the protocol of a BDSM relationship, and any experienced Dom/sub would tell you that. It skips some of the most important processes in building a relationship and the end result of doing that is a lack of trust, at least in the real world of BDSM, and not the movies. That said, there are SOME BDSM relationships that might resemble the plots found in the movie, but they are actually the minority and not the majori-

ty. This form of extremism is not considered an example of good communication in the subculture.

Now before we start getting into specifics on what a Master does, and how he behaves, let's first consider what a Master does NOT do. This is the focus of the next chapter: How to avoid being a Mr. Grey, a Mr. Black or any other exaggerated abusive character, and instead be a true, quality DOM the way your sub wants you to be.

Chapter 3: The Difference Between Abuse and Dominance

Before we start discussing how to act like a real Dom, someone deserving of respect and "worship", let's first spend a little time destroying your INSTINCTS, as most of what you are inclined to want to do—based on misconceptions of BDSM as portrayed by people who don't understand it—are wrong.

A sub experienced in the lifestyle will instantly know if you really understand the "language" or if you're just posing, trying it out because it's the next trendy thing in modern culture.

The first thing to learn about being a master is that it's all about GOOD COMMUNICATION.

Tip #7: Always communicate thoughts to your sub. Everything you say is for communicative purposes. At no time should the slave be confused about what you are saying or what you want.

The sub is not going to bend over backwards to understand you and obey whatever commands you give. By communicating, you establish the power play and you very quickly learn what turns the sub on, and what behavior the sub expects from you.

Patterns of Doms and subs

Tip #8: Follow the game according to the proper formula in order to make sure the slave's emotional, physical and erotic desires are fulfilled.

This basic formula that is similar to any other avenue of sex.

1. Communication and Agreement / Consent

2. Play

3. Aftercare

4. Debrief

For communication, both partners discuss what they want from the experience and from the role play. This is usually the time when strangers get to know each other, and show each other that they are rational, sane and fun-loving people and that they aren't actually psycho killers!

This is also the time where partners discuss limitations and what they absolutely will not do. Safety is discussed, whether that's a "safe word" or simply a discussion of what is off limits beforehand.

This session may be "in character" or may be out of character, but everything spoken should be respected as part of the contract. The agreement phase follows, which is simply reach mutual confirmation of all rules and guidelines.

Next, there is the "scene" or the role play where they are very much in character and breaking taboos—**even while still following the agreements set forth in the first phase**.

The aftercare is necessary because things do get intense during Play, since the Master's intent is to give the sub just as much pleasure-pain as he or she has agreed to endure. Certain "scenes" can be emotionally draining and perhaps physically titillating or slightly painful and so it's quite common for partners to hold each other afterwards so that they can calm down, reconnect, and physically recover – perhaps getting a drink of water or eating.

Next, you have the debriefing, which is almost like an after show to an actor's studio. The participants discuss how the scene went, what they liked about it and what they didn't like about it – constructive criticism so that in the future the scenes will be "just right."

Patterns by Abusers and Masochists

For lack of a better term, we will call people tormented by self-loathing and desiring to be hurt and humiliated, "masochists", since there's not really any other established word for them. The abuser follows an altogether different pattern:

1. Physical or Verbal Disrespect / Aggression

2. Guilt

3. Excuses

4. Apology

5. Planning

6. Set Up

First, the abuser's entire agenda is to brutalize the other partner, whether physically or emotionally. The guilt phase is when the abuser becomes afraid of being caught, exposed, or perhaps losing the partner being abused.

The abuser then goes onto make excuses, justifying his behavior for his abuse. He will usually shift blame, make excuses and rationalize why he must be aggressive and hurtful.

At some point the abuse becomes a burden and the "masochist" will eventually become wise to the antics. At this point the abuser becomes apologetic and becomes the "perfect man", usually becoming a "nice guy", and doing everything the masochists says she wants. Now, the masochist starts to rationalize that he's changing.

The abuser will eventually feel a loss of control and start planning ways to regain it—namely getting away with more abuse and waiting for just the right time and excuse to strike.

The entire motivation is keeping the masochist in a perpetual state of unrest and agitation, making her too afraid to say anything that might upset the abusive lover.

Tip #9: Make sure you rid yourself of all abusive behaviors in action and thought.

It might be instinct for you to take an abusive role, especially if you've never actually read about the complexities of being a Dom. So make sure you're avoiding all traces of tyrannical abuse.

The Effects of a BDSM Master-Slave Relationship

As you can see, real BDSM creates very different emotions in both sub and Dom.

A Master that understands discipline and the psychology of pleasure-pain, as stated mentioned in the formula:

- Uses bodily sensations to create pleasure

- Performs consensual power exchange, so that both lovers feel empowered in their role—even if the sub is "the obedient one"

- The sub is excited to see the Dom
- The Master CREATES trust
- The Master and the slave both feel fulfilled.
- Communication and encouragement between both partners is encouraged.
- The Master follows the "rules" instituted by negotiation in the beginning phase.

In contrast, you'll note that abuse produces emotions of the exact opposite.

- The masochist is injured emotionally or physically
- The sub has no power
- There is no negotiation
- The sub fears the Master and feels anxious in his presence
- All forms of trust are destroyed.

- There is no communication, only the abuser enforcing his will

- The abuser constantly trespasses on boundaries, breaks the rules and gets away with a little more abuse each time, pushing the threshold higher.

Yes, it's sexy to watch a suspense movie like Basic Instinct or Fatal Attraction where one aggressive person constantly pushes someone to the brink of sanity. But that's not what you or your sub are going to want in a real BDSM relationship. Abuse and misogyny are the exact opposite of what real discipline is.

We're going to discuss more about this in the coming chapters, specifically, what you're supposed to be doing rather than abusing your slave.

For now, walk away with this tidbit. Your goal is to have your sub LOVE you, love the discipline you administer, and crave your attention. You don't want a sub that's anxious, crying for help or second-guessing whether or not she's enjoying this.

That's why the BDSM community simplifies the ideology, and does it so well, by saying:

The sub is in control. The Master pleases the sub by giving her the discipline she wants.

Now that misconceptions are out of the way, let's move onto the Role of the Master.

Chapter 4: The Role of the Master

The role of the Master is nothing more than a role, and as we discussed, you discipline, Dominate and sometimes humiliate the sub in just the way she wants. You will often find that "love" is one of the core values of the Dominant/submissive relationship, even if you don't literally "love" your casual sex partner. And as previously stated, not all BDSM relationships involve physical sex. Sometimes it's all about the emotional fulfillment.

The Master, or "Mistress" if a woman takes charge, is named so because the Dom takes ownership rights of the sub—assuming of course that the slave trusts the Dom and the Dom meets their qualifications.

Tip #10: Accept that this is a role you're playing.

It's not necessarily going to be a long-lasting relationships, most likely will not lead to anything romantic in reality, and is a role that you are expected to play well. Method acting, you might say.

Understand that oftentimes, as a Master or Dom, you will be dominating submissives that are not always submissive in other aspects of their life. Some feminists enjoy BDSM role play. Some lovers with control in all other areas of life enjoy the sensation of losing control in the hands of a new partner. They choose to surrender to you, and so the relationship based on trust begins.

Daddy Loves Who He Disciplines

It wouldn't be presumptuous of you to think that many slaves do have "daddy issues", or at least love the idea of a fatherly figure disciplining them in a spirit of love. No, it's not a given in all circumstances and there are plenty exceptions to the cliché. But playing dad (or mom in some cases) as a Dom is a good example to cite, so that we can explain the principles of BDSM.

Tip #11: Learn to love the relationship, the lifestyle and your sub.

It's not love the way you usually think of love, but it's a type of love all new and unique.

In theory, a parent disciplines a child, who is in a lesser role, out of love. The parent invents rules for a child, which are expected to be followed, under threat of punishment.

The submissive party may want to break the rules in order to receive punishment or may simply crave punishment for having already broken the rules. Sometimes the sub doesn't necessarily want punishment but only wants to be told what to do.

What Do YOU Want Out of This?

One thought-provoking question you might want to ask yourself as you plan your new relationship, is, "What do you want out of this?" Since we've already discussed that you're not abusing anyone, nor do you have a license to do so, what attracts about the Dominant role?

Tip #12: Write down your feelings and be honest about what you find erotic.

Imagine what benefit you get from the submissive who interacts with you. You may even think about going beyond the sexual realm and think about lifestyle BDSM—what trust issues do you have and what kind of relationship could help you explore this?

You may not even have thought through what the dominant lifestyle means to you. Did you know, for example, that not all Doms think alike? Some do not subscribe to the notion that the submissive is in charge; the Dom simply reads the submissive's body language or plays by their "archetype" personality, presuming what the submissive wants.

Other Doms are dominant in life, or so they think they are, while other strictly enter a dominant role only in BDSM play, nowhere else. Self-awareness is a very good trait, and knowing what you want from a relationship, and also knowing what you have to give a partner in a relationship. Recognizing your best qualities will help you become a better communicator, and more qualified to take a submissive under your wing.

Now some of being a Dom is common knowledge and a bit simple, and thus easy to comprehend. A dominant partner is confidence, fearless and intensely comfortable with intimacy. He looks into his partner's eyes. He speaks deliberately, with a comfortable volume and with intent to influence his partner's emotions.

Tip #13: Practice speaking dominantly and with a deep internal confidence.

Practice in front of the mirror and see what you look like. Then, practice using this dominant way of speaking with others. You are probably not accustomed to playing this role in reality, since most people would take the Alpha Male face to be a sign of aggression. In the context of BDSM though, it is simply a Master taking on a dominant role. You're not unfriendly, but very assertive. You're calm and comfortable giving orders.

So assuming you have the "look" and the "voice" down, what's next?

What is Leadership?

It's a little basic to say that the dominant "leads" because that's rather obvious. The question is, what is leadership? How do you "guide" the submissive?

The submissive does make it easy, when there's trust, since she (we use the word "she" from now on, for statistical comfort, but obviously he/she is interchangeable) surrenders to the Master's lead, letting him lead the way.

She does not come up with the ideas or lead the conversation. You do. You don't wait to be seduced. You seduce. You take charge.

Tip #14: You cannot be shy or half-hearted about any of this.

You must take charge of the conversation, the encounter and exercise your authority over the sub. Be firm when you speak. And beyond that, always be the one that guides the dialog.

Tip #15: Don't ask her too much.

All a sub really wants to do is give basic answers, perhaps yes or no questions. If you make her think too much, with open-ended questions, she won't be able to focus on the positive feelings this experience brings.

You are also balancing your creativity as a Master, with the rules you establish with your partner at the outset.

Structure and stability are part of leadership, and the benefit that your submissive is getting from all this training and discipline. Whenever you do punish her, it's not because of spontaneous anger or the need to control, as the abuser does; it's with patience and understanding, so that she grows as a submissive—and maybe even as a person. Meanwhile, you also grow stronger and smarter in the lifestyle.

Some believe that a good Master doesn't have to overcompensate by being rude or overly aggressive. He simply "IS", his confidence is internal and his power is felt—no need to prove anything. He commands respect with just a word, or sometimes without a word.

Some BDSM gurus go so far as to say that a Good Master is a **Good Person**, just as a good parent tries to work by a code of ethics. For example:

- Kindness
- Empathy

- Politeness

- Respect

- Honesty

- Ethical Considerations

Tip #16: Constantly check in on yourself, ensuring that you are never doing anything unethical, or anything that the sub doesn't want you doing.

At no point should you lie, intimidate, or disrespect a sub.

Tip #17: A sub may want to be name-called by request, but this is usually not the norm.

Going into this, don't assume that the sub wants you to degrade them. This is a niche-field of BDSM and it's certainly not expected, and will not sit well if you don't discuss it beforehand and just start trash talking.

The basic idea is that if you are these things in life, you will become more naturally and internally confident and thus will not have to adopt a tyrannical personality just to prove your dominance.

Now you may be a bit confused as to how a Dom can take control of a relationship and lead, if he's kind, and if the sub remains in control of the role play. Not to worry, we'll explain more in the coming chapters.

We hope thus far that we've shown the basics of your role as a dominant: loving, strong, powerful and with responsibility as to the welfare of the submissive, who trusts him to keep her safe. This simply isn't possible with a tyrant or an abuser who is constantly putting the submissive in danger.

The role of the Master is to be strong-minded in terms of discipline and training but with the ultimate intent of caring and compassion—to train the sub to do as instructed, in order for the sub to fulfill her wants and needs.

Sometimes you might even talk to subs who will tell you about poor quality Masters they had—men who were merely arrogant and who kept them on a roller coaster ride of despair and anxiety, since that "Master" is ultimately not seeking to please the slave. Only himself, and only in a primitive insecure sort of way.

And if you're a little confused thus far at just what to say and how to act to be a "Good

Master", then it's very important you read the next chapter because this is the second half of understanding your motivation.

What the sub wants.

Chapter 5: The Role of the Slave

This isn't a book on how to play the slave…rather it's how you, as a Master, must understand the slave—the submissive or bottom. Because as we learned, if you want to be an excellent dominant male, qualified to train anyone, then you must learn the personality of the submissive.

Now to some extent, learning the submissive IS a matter of recognizing traditional roles. As in:

- A submissive wants a confident, alpha-male type to tell her what to do

- A submissive trusts you to take care of her, and not push her beyond her comfort zone or beyond what she's ready for in terms of erotic taboos

- A submissive wants to know that you "love" her and that all your discipline is with the intent to help her grow, lead her and train her to obey.

Beyond the peripherals, there is another layer of complexity, and that comes from learning the INDIVIDUAL, and communicating with her.

Now sometimes communication is very explicit and the submissive will tell you exactly what she wants during the "role play", when you will both be in character. However, there are plenty of submissives that STAY IN CHARACTER the whole time and expect you to figure out what they want and how they want to be trained.

We already discussed the important of knowing yourself, your personal strengths and selling points, and now it's time to learn your submissive.

Obviously, *paying attention is vital*.

Tip #18: Make a special effort to listen to your sub, observe her and make mental notes.

Do not be so intent on playing your role perfectly that you don't concentrate on what she is saying and what cues she is giving.

If you focus too much on saying domineering and masterful things…you're going to miss some of her cues and decrease the intensity of the session. Make an effort to:

- Listen to the words she says

- Watching her body language and facial expressions to see what turns her on or makes her stand at attention

- Pay attention to her tone of voice

Once the submissive sees that you are attentive and really making the session all about her taboos and her training, she will start to reveal herself and give you deepest, darkest fantasies for you to fulfill.

That's right—you don't really have to guess at all. You just start communicating, in a relaxed and confident manner.

Some submissives will have a very specific agenda and will not be interested in exploring anything except the niche you spoke about. Some submissives will be all about sex and breaking their own **personal** taboos. Maybe she wants to get in touch with her "inner slut" but is trusting you to let her do so in a safe and strong manner. There are many women who love the idea of exploring their inhibitions, but are afraid to let their desires out without a strong anchor to the real world, at a reasonable level of control, and with full assurances of protection from harm, humiliation or injury.

But reaching this type of intimacy requires that YOU be ready, qualified and responsible.

This brings us to another important point: the submissive does not want to over-think the process. So if your communication doesn't seem to be going well, it's either because you're being domineering rather than dominant, and perhaps you are making her think too much and not FEEL.

Tip #19: Keep your commands, your thoughts and your statements simple. Primal.

Make her feel something by concentrating on emotional communications. Words are secondary compared to the feelings you summon. Even the images you summon in her mind should be based on strong emotion.

Ideally, the submissive wants release, and wants to experience the pain-pleasure associated with this forbidden activity. She wants to essentially turn the rational part of her brain off and SUBMIT to you, knowing that you are going to take care of **the thinking for her**. She wants to feel because of the thoughts you are giving her.

This will be a freeing experience for her, and she can rationalize it away easily, because you are the one in control so all she has to do to unleash her wildest fantasies and desires is submit to you—you who has a plan and will guide her.

What Does the Sub Expect You To Do?

The sub does have some expectations of what you will be doing. In addition to taking the lead and drawing her out in conversation, you may also punish her, train her, give orders and reinforce attitudes through repetition.

What you are actually doing is NOT breaking her rules or pushing her buttons with an intent to hurt or embarrass, but reaching the LIMITS of her boundaries and bending them, **without pushing her too far or over her contract**.

Tip #20: Know what your sub's boundaries are and what behavior would be outside of

her comfort zone — even if the taboo itself is enticing.

You can't really be trusted to protect her if you yourself don't even know what "too far" means. Think in advance of what she does not want and make a clear effort to not surpass this threshold.

Now the sub does expect you to take her outside of her normal routines and do the forbidden things you want to do, and she wants you to do. And she wants you to give her doses of punishment and reward for obeying you or not promptly obeying you.

This intensity is what will keep her coming back to see you.

Power Trade

In order for you to maintain power, and thus continue to have leadership over the sub, you must show pride in yourself, in your desires and speak in a mature voice. This means no apologies, no regrets and no hesitation as to what the command is. This is especially important when speaking your erotic desires aloud. You cannot be shy, or too hesitant to say what you want—since this is part of the turn on, the sub listening to you.

The power trade, you dominating her, only works if there is mutual trust and if she trusts your choices made on behalf of her. This is where training comes into play, because when she learns to trust you is also when you reward her, showing her positive attention and reinforcing this good behavior. This contrasts the "discipline" you give her, at various stages (either for a mistake she made or simply for the kind of person she is).

Tip #21: Don't just punish her. Reward her when she makes an effort to please you.

The give and take, reward and punishment, trains her on how to be a better sub. A reward could be doing something she enjoys (like spanking) or maybe giving her a complement. In contrast, punishment is telling her to do something unfamiliar, perhaps which she feels neutral about. For example, kissing the Dom's feet. This should really be discussed in the negotiation phase because presuming a sub will accept your discipline is presumptuous and could lead to major misunderstandings and a loss of trust.

Honesty Shapes Your Master's Thinking Process

In case you're fretting about what to say and how to say it, just remember this: Honesty always works. Too often, men get flustered trying to say "politely" what they're thinking or trying to phrase an eloquent string of sentences. However, in the "dungeon" of role playing, honesty is the best policy.

There's no reason to lie, and just as in real life, lying only serves to dissolve trust. So don't lie. Instead, make the honesty strong, stark perhaps even what you might call "honest to a fault", the sort of thing you simply wouldn't say in a public conversation.

Being honest with what you want and need from the submissive is a big part of the communication experience and many role players will discuss this before the "scene".

Tip #22: Make it a point to speak honestly and to tell your sub what you're thinking and feeling.

Don't resist saying aloud what you want to say, even if you're socially trained conscience tells you not to.

On the other hand, you are NOT to tell them what you think they want to hear. That's not the truth, and that's not really "honesty", is it?

Honesty is more important than saying the perfect "movie line." It's not about wit or about fast-thinking and speaking. It's about communication. It's about feeling, sensing and "reading" the sub and knowing what they want (by their type), and more importantly, what they're SAYING through verbal and physical cues.

Now how do you avoid hurting the sub's feelings and taking her out of the scene by speaking too honestly?

Tip #23: Don't focus on your own feelings. Focus on what she's feeling. Speak on that. Make this all about what she's feeling, and how her presence makes you feel.

Now that we've discussed the essentials of what the sub wants, and what your motivation is, it's about time to go over the wrong way to execute the RIGHT ideas.

Let's talk about what the mainstream media gets all wrong about discipline.

Chapter 6: The Wrong Way To Do BDSM

Unfortunately, much of what we recognize as BDSM is tainted by an exaggerated and somewhat warped view of domineering behavior, and sometimes bordering on psychopathic emotional abuse. You have since learned what real discipline is and what abuse is…but let's now talk about the wrong way to execute the right idea.

Tip #24: Tell (not ask) your sub what to do. Tell and make sure you let it be known that it is a command.

Wrong Way: Barking orders and being bossy.

Barking orders at the sub totally ignores the context of the arrangement. Since the Dom is doing all of this for the sub's pleasure, it's unrealistic to think that the Master gets to tell the sub what to do all the time. In fact, the sub doesn't owe you any respect or obedience just because you claim to be a Master.

A sub can actually be a very strong, feisty and aggressive person on their own…UNTIL they find a Master that deem mature and wise enough to call their own. This usually means finding someone who understands the complexities of a relationship and the context of the scene.

You earn respect by your actions, by your words and your behavior, always in line with what the sub expects.

Tip #25: Understand that different Doms and subs want different things. Don't jump into play until you research who this person is and what they want.

Wrong Way: Throwing whatever you have on your mind and hoping something sticks.

Dangerous mistake, especially considering how fickle many subs are. Let's face it, it's pretty easy to be a Dom, with all those guys out there thinking this gives them license to be a jerk. It's much more complex to play the part of a sub and to wear your desires nakedly, trusting a Dom to lead you.

So no, you don't want to risk turning her off by throwing a lot of fantasies out at once and hoping she likes something. You owe it to the sub to get to know her. To either talk explicitly about what she wants, or to read her cues.

Know that many subs and Doms have want different things, and sometimes they want very different things at different times. Some are "switch hitters" when it comes to playing Dom and sub. Some want one type of BDSM element from one lover, and a very different element from someone else.

Tip #26: Don't be stubborn. Don't be afraid to change or rethinking your role entirely.

It's practical to remember that if you keep up the Dom side of your personality for years on end, you're eventually going to evolve in the role. The roles do oftentimes change and you won't actually play the exact same character for the rest of your life, even if you have the same life partner. The character changes along with you and your circumstances.

Tip #27: Test her boundaries and help her reach a new plateau of ecstasy. Your intent is to slowly push her to her boundaries giving her just as much as she can take BEFORE overstepping her limits and scaring her.

Wrong Way: Fast-forward to obscenity, orgies, indiscriminate sex and ridiculous, over-the-top challenges.

Another misbehavior is coming on too strong in developing commands and forcing the sub to do something shocking or uncomfortable. It's not your job as the Master to do whatever you want…it's only within the bounds of common sense, not to mention your negotiated contract. A lot of BDSM has excessively mad plot twists involving shocking sex acts performed by a sub all because the Master gained control of her mind.

But in reality, this type of coercion is outside basic common sense, and is certainly not a "safe" thing to do. There goes trust, since the sub is counting on you to be trustworthy.

Tip #28: The sub is going to give you cues so make sure your mind is clear of all distractions and you are concentrating on her level of communication.

Wrong Way: So I'll just wait till the sub tells me what to do, right?

Way off! Even though the subs do know their role and your role, it may surprise you to know that some subs actually lie to you, attempt to throw you off as a test. Others may actually be ignorant as to what they want or need and perhaps will only have a vague idea of what they want to happen.

If this is the case, you do LEAD, you handle the relationship responsibly, above all making sure they remain safe and in good physical and emotional health.

Tip #29: Think of it as a dance, where the man leads and the woman follows. This way, there are not two people leading and confusing the steps.

The Dom starts with conversation and action and the sub follows the Dom's lead, complementing the progress of thought.

Many slaves actually carry around the viewpoint that they would not be subservient to just anyone, and some dominant men similarly think they would not want to be Master over just anyone, just because they "could." It takes a special connection. A process of understanding, negotiation and equal trade.

One really has to look into a sub's heart and mind to see their desires, their passions, and fantasies for what they are—the psychology behind it, and perhaps even the vulnerability.

Tip #30: Realize that being a Master is a learning experience. You will learn and you will get better as you go along. Stay strong and determined.

Wrong Way: Whoops, I messed up. Let's start over. Or let's just laugh it off.

Mistakes are a mood-killer, plain and simple. Now that doesn't necessarily mean flubbing a word or losing your train of thought is unforgivable. But losing your CONFIDENCE and laughing about it is unacceptable. The Master must be in control of the scene AT ALL

TIMES and must not surrender that leadership role until the aftershow and debriefing phase.

Just get it through your head that mistakes are not an option. It's better to practice, to come up with better reactions than totally losing your sub's focus and the intensity of the moment. Work hard on perfecting your voice, your look, your calm demeanor and your high self-esteem. Don't let HER see YOU sweat. This means you surrender power to her and that is the exact opposite of what must happen.

Think of it like the boss at work who can never let his employees know that he's nervous or struggling. The minute the employees sense it they lose respect. It's much the same in a fetishistic relationship where control and the illusion of leadership means EVERYTHING. Don't take the trust she gives you for granted. This isn't just a game. This is a lifestyle choice.

And yes, it is true that the sub ultimately controls the relationship, but…

Tip #31: The Master controls the SCENE. The scene is what you create and you must totally control all aspects of it, shaping the setting yourself.

In the next chapter, we're going to move onward into what BDSM should be—namely a personal mission. A way to make peace in your mind. Your world, your fantasy, in which everything you've ever desired comes true.

Chapter 7: What Creates a Personal Taboo?

BDSM has to be personal, or else why is it erotic? The pleasure and pain scale that you endure means nothing unless it titillates you, and usually titillation comes from a very personal and profound reaction to stimuli.

Let's face it, if you don't have a foot fetish, a person licking your toes won't do much for you, even if you laugh and try to enjoy it. BDSM is all about having a very intimate connection with a partner and an intense shared experience.

We would be remiss if we didn't refer back to the Freudian theory that many fetishes are the result of childhood issues, perhaps trauma, or sometimes simply a genetic attraction to some type of person, behavior or thing. According to one study, many respondents stated that their realization of a BDSM fetish started before the age of 15, so it develops early and is intrinsically related to developing sexuality.

When going on your own personal adventure in taboo eroticism, first determine if there is a particularly idea or thought that turns you on, or if you want to discover new thoughts that sound appealing.

Tip #32: Start by admitting what your own turn ons are and trace them back to childhood, adolescence and onward.

Examine what situations led to these "anchors" or "triggers" that make you feel passionate. Is it the loss of control? Or is it something more tangible and sensual that made you feel safe? Even though you are not playing the sub, being aware of what causes these kinks in the first place will only help you.

Not all subs know what they want, and so you as the Master may want to discuss ideas with them during the negotiation, or perhaps during the scene itself, as long as you take it slow and according the sub's comfort level.

One common practice in sex therapy is to have couples go through a list of acts, some of which might be taboo, just to have one partner veto the idea or leave it on the "maybe" category. If you find that you or the sub have never really thought about forbidden fantasies, then going through a list of what other people find erotic, repugnant or intensely "wrong" might be a starting point.

This will at least help you become accustomed to the idea of experimentation. And sometimes you don't even know if you like something or if your partner does, until after experiencing it for the first time.

Tip #33: Create your own list and figure out where you stand on some of these acts and just what is too far for you.

Doing this, and realizing your own limitations, is a good way to know yourself and eventually become better at learning what another person wants, needs, and can handle. (Sometimes, believe it or not, you know better than they do if they can handle something)

Don't be surprised or ashamed if and when you realize that certain fetishes are traced back to early development. However, not everyone is in agreement as to why they develop so early and what set of circumstances influence the behavior.

What does seem to be universally accepted is the idea that we establish boundaries in our youth and immediately perceive an idea that is wrong, morally and ethically. We then tend to carry that attitude throughout our lives; hence, while we remain opposed to the idea because of instinct and a trained conscious, the temptation to try the taboo, whether due to suppressed passion or just curiosity of the unknown, becomes more intense.

As a child a person explores his or her world, their shaping attitudes and morals, through playing, testing and learning. In adulthood, sex is much the same way. The person latches onto an idea that feels instinctively dangerous or wrong and then he or she is SLOWLY exposed to it, allowing the person to surrender to the taboo and lose control. The Master takes control.

In this other "world", an alternate world of performance, the sub can let someone take her on a journey, to the boundaries, to the brink of their deepest, darkest unfulfilled fantasy.

This enticing concept, this forbidden pleasure (a little scary, just as it's sensual) is what leads to greater orgasms, in terms of multiples, or more intense singles. Your mind is involved and your mind is the most important organ to stimulate. All the other toys and techniques used in BDSM, including the imagery and the painful or sensual accessories you buy, is just supporting the erotic thought that starts the process.

Tip #34: Identify the THOUGHT, the taboo, that is actually turning your partner on.

It's not simply, a roomful of toys or a dungeon with restraints. What thought is fueling the desire? What's the thought that is strong enough to make the sub submit to all these toys, scenarios and captivity settings? Identity the thought before you go on with creating a scene.

How Much of Erotic Desire is Social?

To some extent, BDSM is about rejecting the traditions and constraints of society. In the book *"A Billion Wicked Thoughts: What the World's Largest Experiment Reveals About Human Desire"*, the authors research the importance of an erect penis as a one of the most important demonstrations of male virility, aggression, marking territory, and male-to-female courtship.

In some instances, the very primitive instinct of sperm competition amongst men is believed to cause cuckolding fantasies. One theory is that if another man has sex with a taken woman, the cuckold party sometimes feels compelled to have intercourse with her afterwards, with more forceful and aggressive contact, and will thus deposit more sperm volume—as if proving himself superior to the other male.

As you can see, fetishism and erotic taboos can be socially nurtured or personally meaningful.

Tip #35: Try identifying some of your own socially nurtured taboo fetishes, that is, fantasies that are not necessarily personal but still exciting because of the social taboo.

For instance, public sex is something a lot of people would like to try, only because society deems it is inappropriate. Learning of some common fantasies, nurtured by a condemning society, will help you better learn the mind of a sub.

Naturally, corporal punishment is one of the first touching experiences students have in school, and it's not so uncommon that they develop erotic feelings towards spankings, as this past trauma eventually becomes an imprint on the psyche, sparking feelings of forbidden pleasure-pain associations.

The very idea of "sinning" or transgressing against a moral or social code is typically exciting because of the danger, and yet these desires—usually base and animalistic—are relegated to fantasy scenes in our own mind (or a BDSM dungeon) because they are literally too dangerous to try in reality, and certainly among people whom we just met and have no relationship with. Essentially, it's the fear of society turning on us that creates the taboo attraction.

As far as BDSM goes, it is commonly believed that one reason why some men do prefer submission fantasies is because of social conditioning that suggests men have to be dominant. And thus, a lot of what we see in experimental BDSM involves men who are "turned into" women. Again, going against all social traditions and picking at our insecurities—as a civilization and as individuals, with unique memories.

Tip #36: If you're the Dom, you really have to understand BOTH your role and the sub's role, including what the sub wants from the relationship.

You have to be empathetic, and actually feel what the sub feels, knowing how to satisfy her completely—giving her the pain and pleasure she craves.

It's not surprising then that some Doms are "switchers" and capable of playing Dom or sub, only because they understand both roles intimately.

So it's safe to say that talking things out is the best way to find your taboo. Or if you're a perceptive Dom, watching the sub to learn what makes her tick, and what she's saying with her body language and eyes. It's a simple process of discovery, and one that you can always adapt to, improve and fall back, if necessary.

Of course, once you identify the "taboo" it quickly becomes a matter of learning the limits and boundaries, just as important to this puzzle as the taboo itself. This is the subject of our next chapter.

Chapter 8: Learning Yourself and the Sub's Limits

Here's a common problem you see in fake BDSM, or movie-style BDSM which is highly sensationalized. A shy and suppressed woman (a sub in training) admits her attraction and then gets seduced into a world of erotic thrills by the Dom who fulfills her fantasies. The problem is, that Dom is moving too fast. There's also no communication, no indication that the sub is ready to move forward for more intensity. The Dom simply presumes she's ready. And perhaps realistically, the story ends on a sour note—the sub has suffered too much and is now traumatized by the ordeal.

That's something to think about. **If you move too fast you will scare the sub away**. You will violate the trust and she will leave, since as we already discussed, the sub has the power to end the relationship if you disregard the contract. If the relationship has become one-sided and abusive, the sub really gets nothing out of it.

Therefore, although obviously you have your own limits as to what you can do, the SUB's limits are the primary consideration. It's true that you should make your own list of do and do nots because it's always a better idea to discuss this beforehand than to run into complication during the "scene", when you're both in character. Ideally, safe words are just "emergency" fallouts, since if you respect the contract and the agreements made beforehand, the situation shouldn't reach the point where the sub feels unsafe.

Therefore, after deciding what is within your limitations, it's time to focus on what's in the sub's limits, and what is beyond the boundaries of what they can endure. Too much of a good thing, even if it's something you like, can be downright traumatic and painful in the not-so-fun way.

Think of it like eating a dessert you like. You may crave that dessert hungrily, for the entire day perhaps. But eating too much of it will make you sick.

Or think of it in terms of dating. You like somebody. But instead of taking it "slow", your crush immediately begins stalking you, harassing you and making all sorts of demands of your time. Suddenly, what was once exciting is now **horrifying**.

This is especially true in BDSM lifestyle.

Tip #37: Your ultimate goal is to take the taboo and reach a peak of erotic fulfillment, but you must do it slowly.

If you don't, it will be more than the sub can endure and it will turn from pleasurable to painful to excruciating torture. So taking it slow is obviously the first step.

Communication is vital, and this refers to ongoing communication, since it will actually take more than one conversation, and perhaps more than one session to build trust. Therefore, you never push the sub beyond the trust she has for you. If you just started the relationship, trust is not going to be that strong—you simply can't move too quickly.

Being True to Yourself

This is actually very important as you must be realistic with yourself long before you start talking to your sub. Are there things you are not comfortable doing? Then don't pretend. More to the point…

Tip #38: Don't pretend to be another kind of Dom that you saw in a movie.

Just because you see someone else doing it doesn't mean it's right for you. Most people that do really amazing things and put on a good performance are very experienced. They've studied and practiced. Don't measure yourself with someone's model; develop your own UNIQUE style. Being introspective and realizing your strengths is pivotal. Ignore whatever is trendy and stick to what you know.

It also helps to figure out what type of Dom you want to be and spend all your time working towards that. Believe it or not, not all Doms act the same. There are various types, different personalities, and ways of dealing with subs. So it's a great idea to add your own personal style to the scene.

Also, understand that many in the BDSM community find it ostentatious to create a title for yourself, especially if you're just starting out. It may actually cause people to laugh, since few people go around calling themselves "Master" or "Mistress", certainly not in reality, and not even in BDSM—at least not when you just start.

It might help to discover who you really are, and the Master you want to be, by creating your own title, one that fills you with confidence and that is unique. Choose something that other people will respect, nothing too over the top, since you're obviously not going for humor here, nor self-aggrandizement.

Tip #39: Start thinking of your personal strengths, since these will be your greatest assets as a Dom—not simply pretending to be something you're not.

What qualities of strength do other people see in you and admire about you? How can you turn these ordinary good qualities into something powerful and dominant for your alter ego of Master?

What qualities do you value most about yourself—perhaps intelligence, patience or creativity? Maybe your looks, your voice or your charm are your greatest assets. Don't throw away these good points trying to be someone else. Use them to your advantage.

Keeping it (Not) Real

Tip #40: It is strongly recommended that you only form relationships with subs that you know fairly well and are in good terms with in "reality."

Any negativity and awkwardness is going to slow you down or cause trust issues, and sometimes meeting a stranger for the first time is awkward.

Before embarking on a BDSM journey, it is best to establish trust in the "real world".

For example, telling your sub that she should tell someone else where she is going and who she is going to be with. You don't have to tell them the purpose of the visit, but let them feel safe by having this protection put in place. You can also do the same for yourself, having your own contact, and let the sub know. This instantly creates trust.

Tip #41: Are you making precautions for your BDSM play, making sure the sub has everything she needs to feel safe and cared for?

Being smart and compassionate in this regard is not a mistake.

Most Masters will have a first aid kit on hand, as well as any other precautions in case of an emergency like a flashlight or a fire extinguisher. Some even learn CPR just in case of a breathing problem, choking or fainting.

Tip #42: Don't drag your personal life into the scene.

Even if you are upset about something in reality, that negative energy can upset the balance of a trusting BDSM encounter.

This is why most Doms will not play if they are in a bad mood, or if the sub is in a bad mood. There is more risk in this case. Even drug use will probably disqualify you to make judgment and being someone's Dom is all about making good judgment calls.

Since in a way, BDSM is art, it's not wise to mix reality with the art. Don't bring up anything from the real world into the "scene", as if punishing someone for something in the real world. It takes the sub out of the experience and will not do much for strengthening trust.

The Agreement Phase

So much of the initial communication will be done in the agreement phase before the scene starts. Negotiate with each other, always aware that there are some things the sub will not want you to do, and maybe vice versa. You need to consider such aspects of the encounter as:

- Behavior allowed
- Safe sex requirements
- Degree of bondage/pain

Any limitations on physical or emotional stressing

Tip #43: It's safer to take it slow and work towards a long-range goal of absolute ecstasy.

If you take it too slow, you can always make the next session better. If you make it too hard or fast early on, you can easily lose trust and destroy the whole relationship.

The Debriefing Phase

After the scene and the after care, you will communicate again. The sub will tell you what about the scene she liked and anything she didn't like. The questioning phase for yourself goes beyond the debriefing. You will ask yourself why you do the things you do, why it worked, and how to improve. Self-criticism is not easy but it is very important if you want to grow as a Dominant.

Tip #44: Keeping an open mind is crucial, as there may be a lot of delicate "dynamics" in certain relationships, or perhaps desires that a sub has.

You really only have two choices. You either go along with it, or walk away saying it's not for you. There is no in between. You can't half-heartedly play a scenario, nor can you whine, complain or mock the scenario. That's a violation of trust. Having empathy for the other person is always the aim of a good Dom and knowing what they want is part of being a good Dom.

Now that we've discussed the fundamentals of being a good Dom, let's "zoom out" and get a little broader. You understand the personal aspect of being a Dom. Now let's consider the emotional and social aspect of domination and what the sub expects you to do.

Chapter 9: Creating Gut Level Attraction by Unleashing Your Passions

Ideally, BDSM works because you are stripping away intellect and social standards that inhibit raw attraction. Essentially, we are animals and we respond like animals to basic human behavior; our social standards is what keep us in check, making sure we balance our primitive instincts to mate and dominate with rationality and respect.

For instance, consider sexual roles in society today. We live in age of post-feminism, one where women more or less do get a fair shake at the career they want and the type of relationship they want—although things are not completely fair yet, obviously. Still, our social etiquette suggests that liberated women should be treated with respect and deference.

In the BDSM world, we strip away the pretenses of polite behavior and respectful treatment. Instead, it's about attraction, dominance and assertive behavior. Not aggressive. Violence done onto the submissive is not enough, and in many cases, is not requested at all. Instead, the Dom controls and guides the sub, treating them like a submissive spouse or perhaps even a child, depending on what type of dynamic is requested. It's too simplistic to say, "I want the Dom to abuse me or be rough with me." A more accurate explanation would be, "I, as the sub, want to be protected, loved, disciplined, cherished, and rewarded."

Tip #45: The strength of the Dom is what turns the sub on and keeps in a willing state of subservience.

The Dom is not "equal to the sub", as is politically correct (PC) to say. The Dom is stronger, wiser and superior. He knows what's best for the sub and the belief she has in him is what gives her the courage to follow through and a direction in life (or this alternate life).

You could say that the desire to dominate a partner is instinctive and not at all what we actually do in respectable PC society. The

BDSM Master role is comparable to the old concept of Men presiding over the household, having wives in subjection, just as he does the children. What he says goes and his role is firmly established. Oftentimes, all he has to do is say a word to demand the respect and adherence of his wife or child.

You see, when a Dom is in control there is no need to bully, degrade or rough up a partner. If a partner wants those things, then that's a different story. But in terms of creating gut level attraction, all what is necessary is for the sub to have the right frame of mind. He is in control. He is dominant. He doesn't have to prove anything. The sub, turned on and feeling protected by him, will willingly submit to his authority.

Another interesting tidbit: subs are not naturally self-loathing. They don't want EVERYONE to dominate them and this distinguishes them from Authentic Masochists who really do want people to mistreat them. No, a real sub is sure of herself, proud of who she is, and really will only submit to a man she deems worthy of her subservience. So it's not just, "I am a woman (or sub) and I need a man to control me." It's more along the lines of "I need someone strong enough to handle me."

Submission is brought upon by the ...ing of trust.

Remember that above all else, because so many new masters forget this and try to bully their way to Master. But in actuality, the sub gives the "GIFT" of submission to a man who earns it. It is a commitment and a responsibility.

How Does the Master Guide the Scene?

The next question to ask is, attitude aside, what does the Master actually do to guide a scene? The Master is in charge of creating and "directing" the scene, according to the specifications of the sub. This is important because if the sub were to come up with the scenario, she would be in control. Relocating to a different scene is essential in surrendering control.

The Master is still creating the scenario for the slave, and is ultimately helping the slave to embrace the taboo attraction. If he does his job right the slave will want to do everything and the Master will not have to demand anything.

The slave craves authority and so always maintaining that authority is necessary, and much of this is determined by the slave herself. If she wants to be disciplined she will let him know and he will administer it. If she is already submitting to his authority, she will obey him.

Tip #47: It's interesting to note that by the time the slave is ready to enjoy the experience, submission has already happened.

A slave cannot reach the next state while still fighting the authority or asking for discipline. The Master must have trained the slave by now, making sure trust is stronger than ever. Because the next phase is called the "trance" or sometimes "Subspace".

This is an ecstatic state of mind, where erotic desire is heightened by exploring the taboo and then tension is released. It is an altered state of mind, one where rational thinking dissipates and the slave simply has to obey and feel everything the Master is telling her. All distractions are let go and the slave simply feels the intensity of the moment.

So now you know the basic formula for the scene as well as the end goal. **Training, gaining complete trust, and then Subspace**. Your goal is to take your sub by the hand and guide them through this process.

The Importance of Practice

Practice makes perfect—you've heard that, right? It definitely applies here because you can't expect to be a Dom by simply reading about it. It takes life experience, BDSM experience, and personal experience, just like any other subject.

Tip #48: Talk to other Doms in the lifestyle and ask them questions. Get more specific and personal experience as to how they play the role and how they deal with a wide variety of subs. You can find a mentor in the lifestyle, whether you only want to be a Dom or want to be a Switcher, playing both Dom and sub.

Some Doms, unwilling to be trained by someone else, find it useful to create a group of friends for advice, or perhaps join a forum. This helps to ensure that they are getting information from other sources, and not limiting their viewpoints to their own instincts.

Practice may also encompass a bold experiment.

Tip #49: You may want to actually undergo training as a sub, just to feel what it's like.

They always say that before you burden someone with a task, you ought to do it yourself, so that you can always keep your empathy. Nothing will help you better in gaining empathy than by subjecting yourself to the same treatment you plan to give others. You will very quickly learn that brutality is not what you want, or want someone else wants.

It's also important to remember that you will mess up occasionally, whether it's forgetting something, misspeaking, or breaking character. It's bound to happen at first, and as you gain experience it will happen less frequently. But even experienced Doms do make mistakes.

All you can do is accept the mistake and then move forward, quickly, not staying in the moment and feeling negative about it. Instead of trying to "fix" the mistake, you simply disregard it. But you learn from it later on, as you think it over and realize where you went wrong. Incorporate your notes into the next scene.

Now this does NOT mean that you just pretend you did nothing wrong and that everything you do is perfect. Don't lie. Never lie or feed your own ego by breaking trust. Making the sub feel bad for your mistake does NOT create trust. This is a relationship based on trust, not a tyranny that thrives on fear.

Tip #50: Always take responsibility for who you are, the role you are playing and all decisions you make.

Lying to yourself or your sub will not save face. A real Dominant Master has nothing to hide.

How about the tricky issue of apologies? Isn't it safe to say that you should never apologize if you are in a scene? True, you don't break character and apologize. However, if you ever sense that you have hurt your sub or gone beyond what was negotiated, in the debriefing phase where you return to reality, it may be prudent—if the sub is feeling upset about it.

If the sub is happy and clearly indicates that she liked where you went with the scene, obviously there is no need to apologize. You don't apologize for what you both want, what this is, and what your unique relationship involves, even if it's incomprehensible to someone on the outside. You both accept it.

In our final chapter we're going to discuss another complex topic—BDSM as a form of therapy. Yes, you heard that right. At its best, BDSM lifestyle is more than just a game or a way to get your rocks off. It's a form of healing.

Chapter 10: BDSM as Surrogate Therapy

You might be surprised at how seriously people take BDSM—not merely as a form of sexual play, but as an honest to goodness form of therapy.

Some people will tell you that they turned to the lifestyle at a point of desperation in their lives, perhaps by accident, or even figuring they have nothing left to lose. This was certainly the case for one "retired" BDSM Switcher who gave an interview for this book, under the request of anonymity, and revealed something very important about the motivations of Doms and subs. Mistress X spoke candidly about the experience, stating it was a turning point in her life—even now, when she has moved passed the practice.

Q: Why did you stop practicing the lifestyle?

A: Because I didn't need it anymore. I got out of it what I wanted. It was something I desperately needed at the time. I was seriously spinning out of control and holding on as tight as I could. I had a life of hell. I lost a relative very close to me, my fiancé, my family wasn't speaking to me, and I had various medical problems. I was spinning completely out of control. I was either drunk or jacked up on drugs. I couldn't cope. One day I wound up meeting a Dom. He knew in an instant I was in need of help. I was at the point where I didn't care about anything, including the risks I was taking. He knew I was going through a hard time and made it his job to take care of me. He loved helping people. He was and is a beautiful man.

Q: How did he treat you?

A: He didn't play daddy or train me. My Dom took complete control of me. He had my list of what I didn't want. For someone like me, that has trouble dealing with emotions, this relationship was the perfect way to release them. It strips everything else away and leaves you with just your primal self. People, like me, who are under the weight of so much emotion and can't process it, want to be completely dominated.

Q: Can you explain the concept behind pleasure and pain?

A: It's a fine line between pain and pleasure...that's the lesson you really learn. The pain is similar to why people cut themselves. You learn how to take your pain and make it pleasurable...how to not fear it. While you're feeling physical pain, you're obliterating emotional pain. If you think about the developmental parts of our lives, the way children learn through play and imitation...this is like the grown up version of that. And more often than not, it's completely not sexual. It's a very effective way of processing emotions.

In conversing with the retired Mistress, we see what is at the heart of BDSM, and why, in one sentence, that so many people get the culture and lifestyle wrong.

It's about processing emotion and not just sexual gratification.

That alone tells the story. BDSM is a way to express yourself sexually as a Dom, or reconcile sexual feeling as a sub. And you will find that as you keep going and reaching new peaks of ecstasy and discovery, that you will reach a peak that goes beyond just sexual fulfillment. It will feel cathartic, maybe even something comparable to therapy.

Now we're not saying it is "legitimate therapy", to be confused with actual medical-licensed therapy. Certain emotional and mental problems can only be resolved with a doctor's supervision. However, for body issues, sexual issues, erotic taboos, and even what you might call "closure" for past mistakes in your life, it really can help you to reconcile buried feelings and turn a lot of inward pain into outward pleasure.

It's a very Freudian approach to "therapy", that's for sure. And no doubt, Freud's aggressive and intimate techniques are no longer considered professional behavior. In the same way, you could say that BDSM lifestyle is an alternative, "underground" and off the record form of emotional healing. Proponents of the lifestyle confess it's a much more hands-on approach to addressing sexual and lifestyle problems that they really can't get from mere "advice" or "counseling." In that way, it would be comparable to sex surrogacy, escort service, and other "fringe" career choices that are not mainstream, but still very much appreciated by people who actually investigate the process and personally go through the experience.

You, as the Dom in training should be eager to learn all you can from others who have lived the lifestyle and have much wisdom to offer. Don't close your mind to new ways of looking at things. Don't assume that BDSM is all attitude and no research because frankly, the opposite is true.

It's doing the research and learning your sub. Your attitude comes natural once you recognize who your sub is and what they want/need from you.

This really is an art form all about helping other people through more unorthodox means. Therefore, you can understand why depictions of BDSM, usually associating the lifestyle with danger, disrespect and psychosis, are completely wrong and do more damage than good.

BDSM is everything you want it to be. It's sexy, taboo and certainly not "vanilla" in any respect. It's "extreme" in the sense that it's not just sex, not just therapeutic and not just being "nice." It's a little bit of everything and that's why it does require a guide. It's complex, yes. But once you understand the fundamentals you will be better able to improvise and find your unique voice.

After a final word, we're going to share with you some other need-to-know information that will be of great interest to you as you continue your Dom training.

Conclusion

We hope you have taken the advice to heart and are ready to try your new role out for size, always making sure that your sub is happy, protected and disciplined in the way a Dom should properly administer discipline.

Let's admit it…this lifestyle is not getting a very good review from the mainstream media because of all the misunderstandings. Sadly, there are still many pretender Doms out there who think BDSM is all about abuse, barking orders and acting like a jerk. They are totally oblivious of the concepts of BDSM, the history, the psychology and the "healing" factor that it really takes into account.

We hope that if you are really interested in going through Dom training that you will be one of the Good Doms and will serve as a good example of the way Doms really are.

You can help other people in this lifestyle. You can also teach people the value of this training and how it can be a source of strength and recovery for people who are reaching out to their fellow man for loving care.

You've already discovered a part of this puzzle—namely becoming the Dom that a sub wants. However, you still have much to learn about the art of Dominating itself. In volume 2 & 3 in this series, we will discuss:

- How to talk like a Dom

- How to create a "scene" that keeps her attention

- Where to find a partner

- Games and toys that can help

- How to reach the "trance" state so that the sub feels all the ecstasy she wants

- And more.

Until our paths cross again, keep safe, keep it positive and always keep an open mind.

Manufactured by Amazon.ca
Bolton, ON